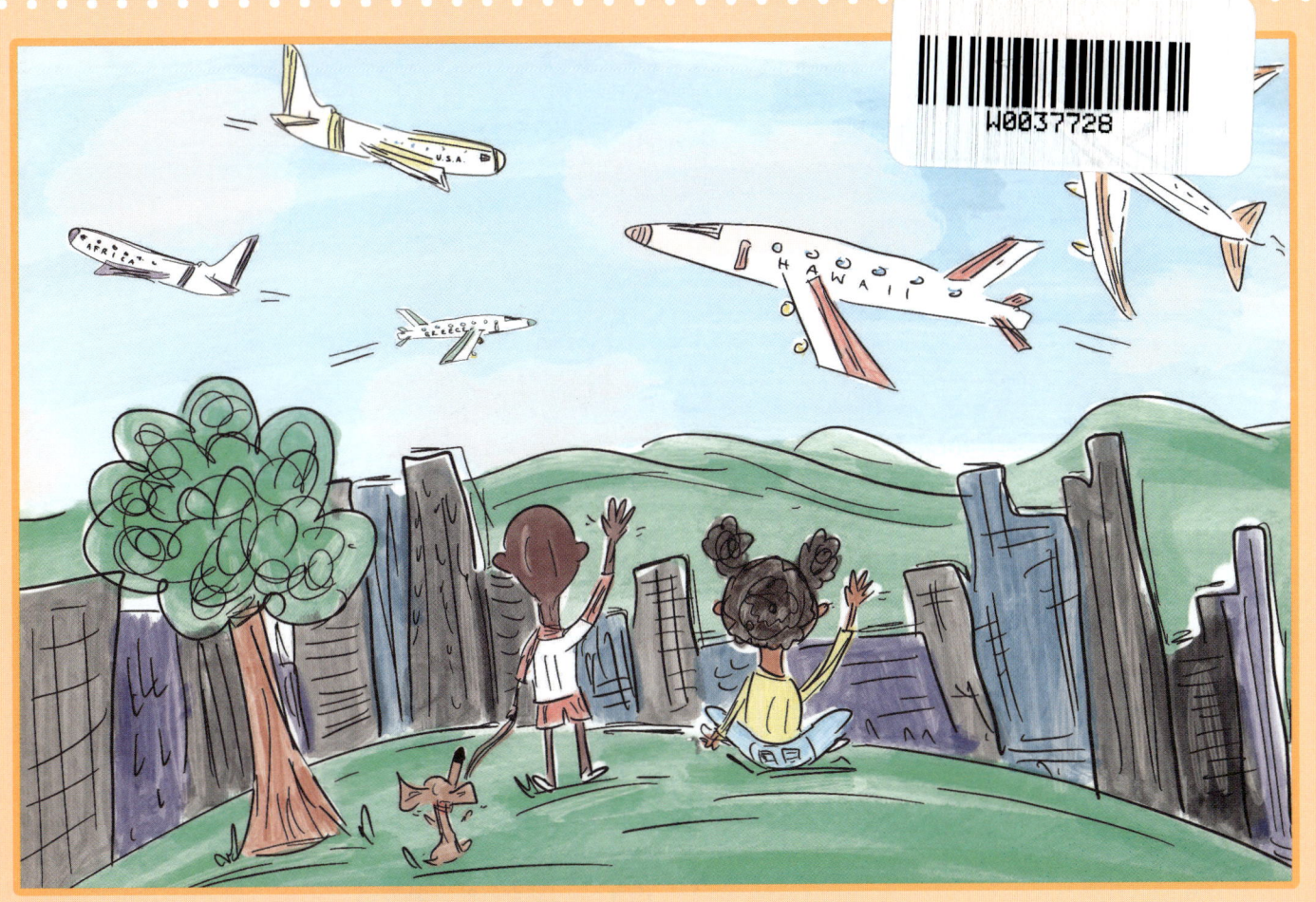

Hi! I'm Anthony. My favorite place in the whole world is a hill by the airport. Silly I know! But I love to sit there and watch the planes take off. Traveling all over the country. All over the world! Bringing people and packages to all sorts of places! My sister drives us there every day after school. We spend hours and hours watching the planes as they shoot off into the sky.

1

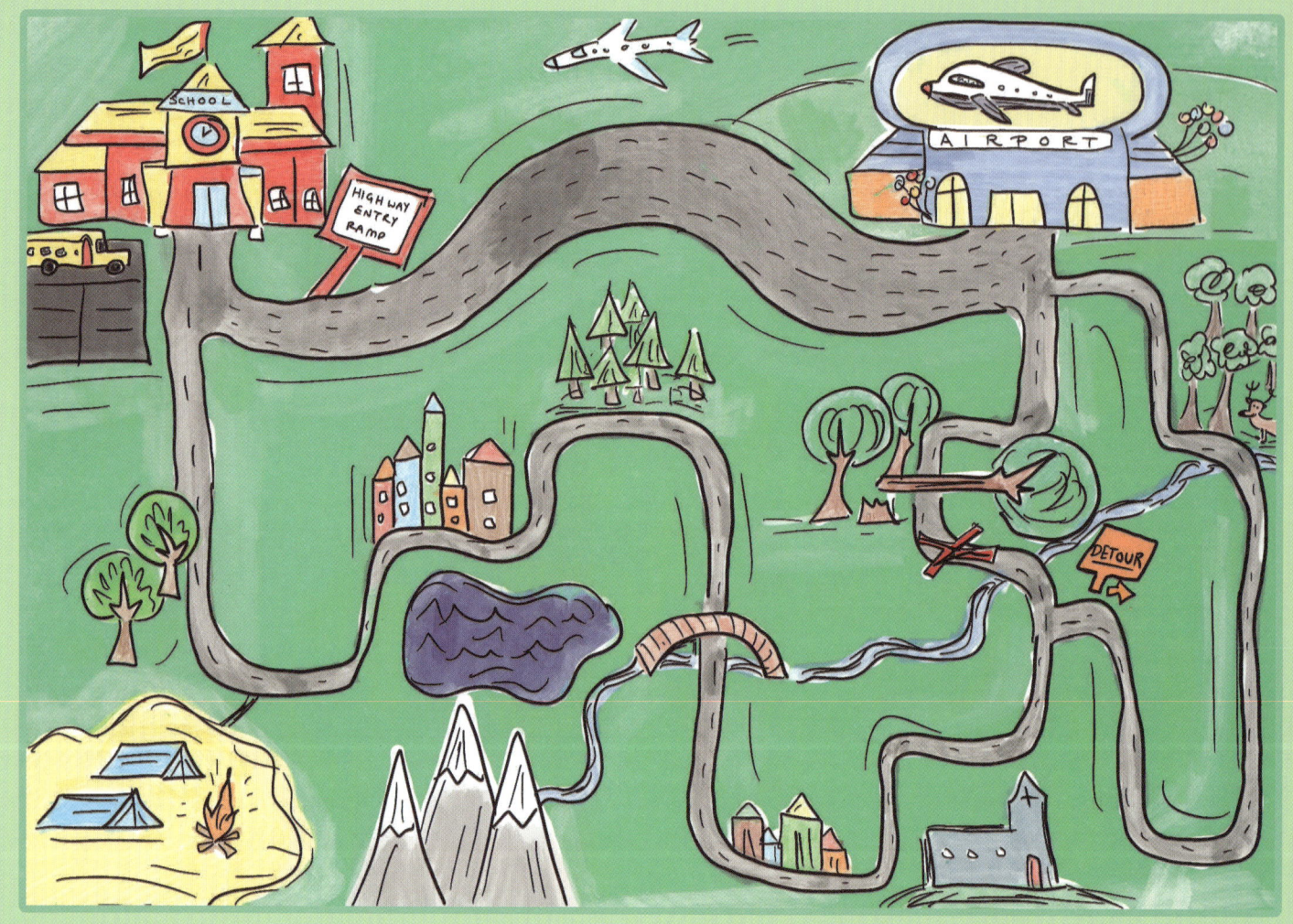

Unfortunately, Mom says we always have to be home by dinner time. So, we better get there as fast as we can after school to have as much time as possible! On our first trip, my sister and I looked at a map to plan the fastest route. There were two different routes we could take. The backroads or the highway.

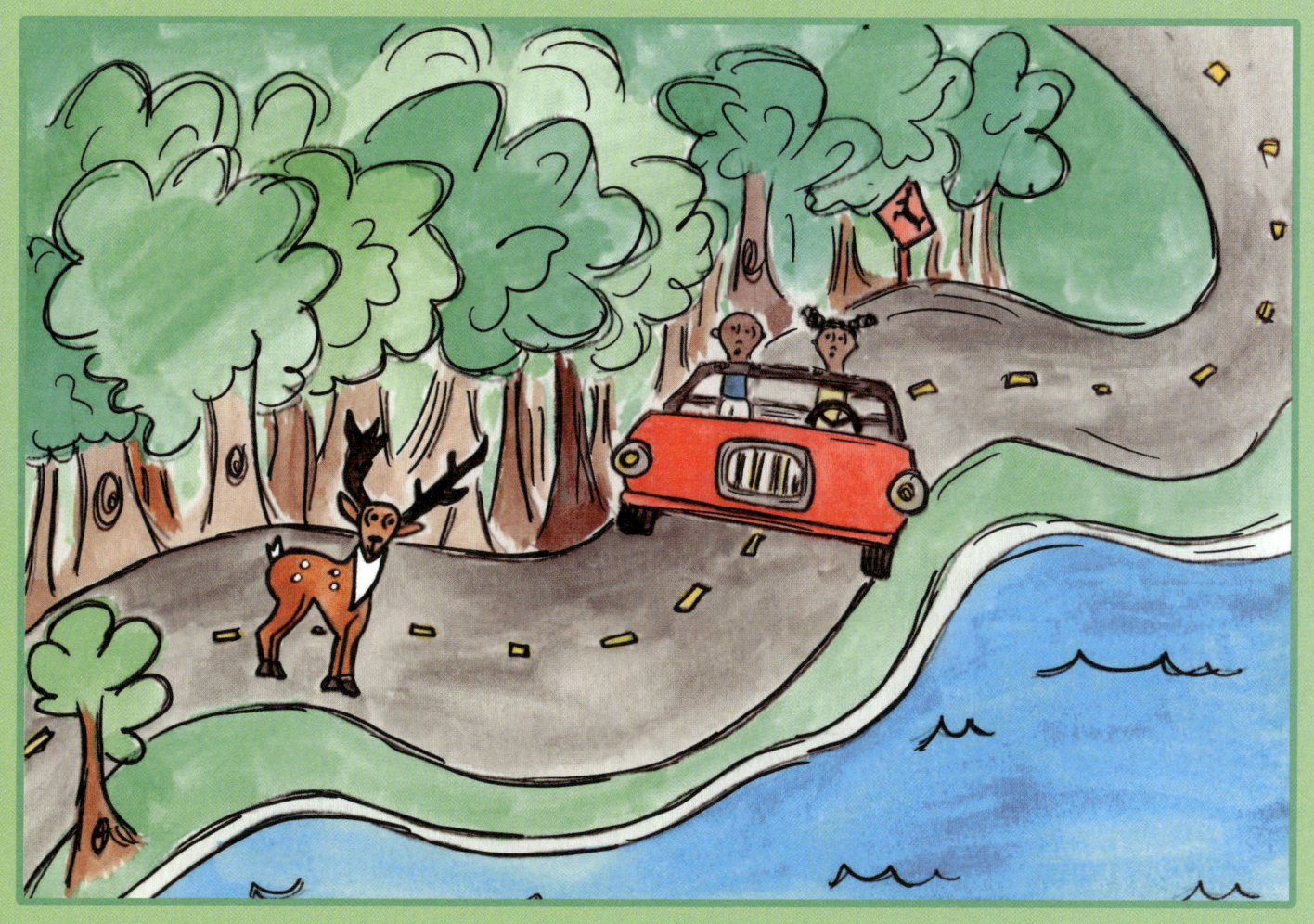

First, the backroads. These are teeny, tiny roads. They branch and wind. We hit detours. Sometimes the roads are broken. And bumpy. Sometimes they're blocked by trees and we have to turn around. Sometimes deer are crossing, and we have to wait. Sometimes we get lost and never even make it to the airport!

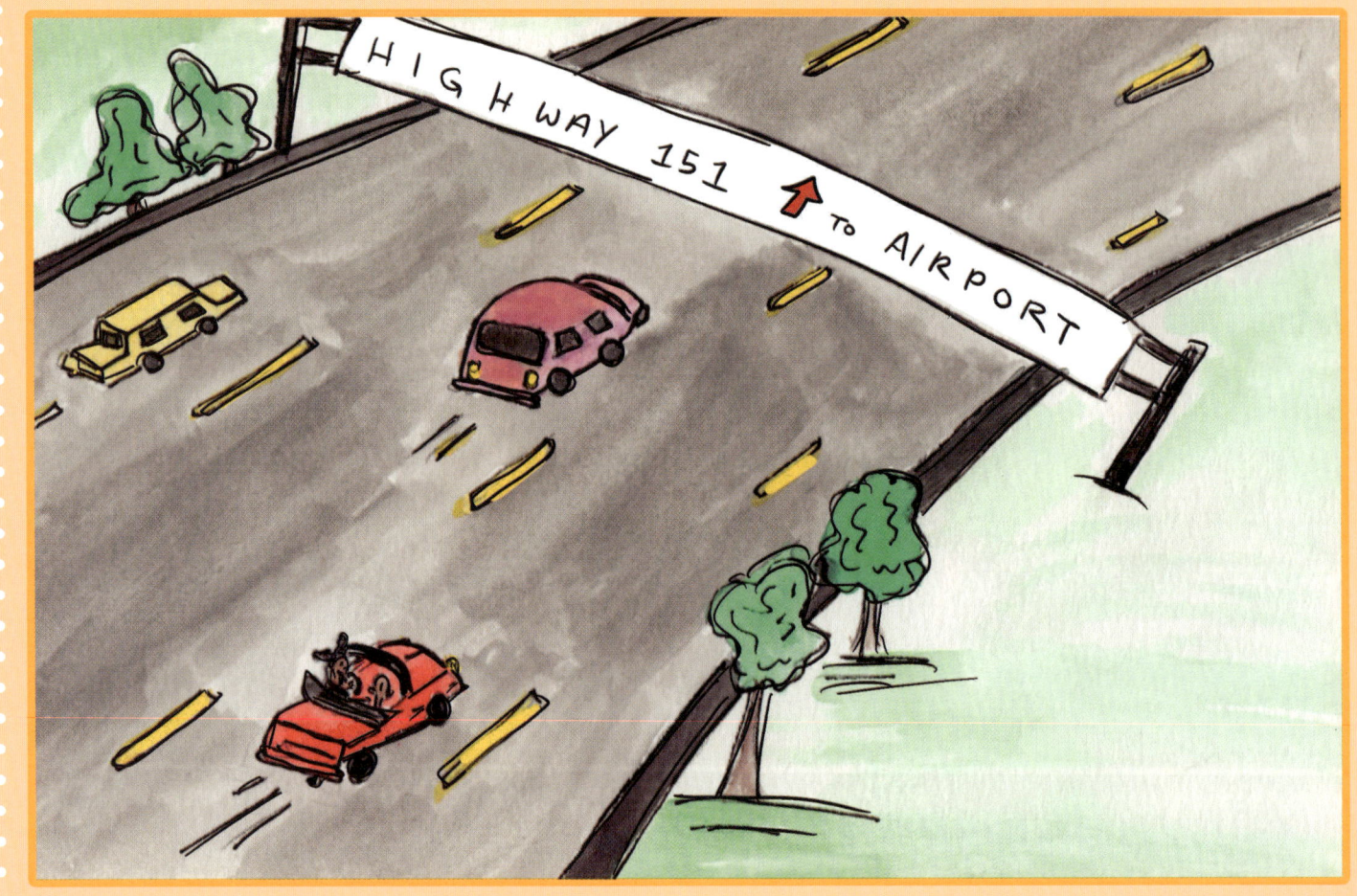

Then there is the main highway that takes you right where you want to go. The magical highway. We jump right on and shoot straight to the airport. We get there so fast (and not just because my sister drives fast...)

It is definitely the best route to take!

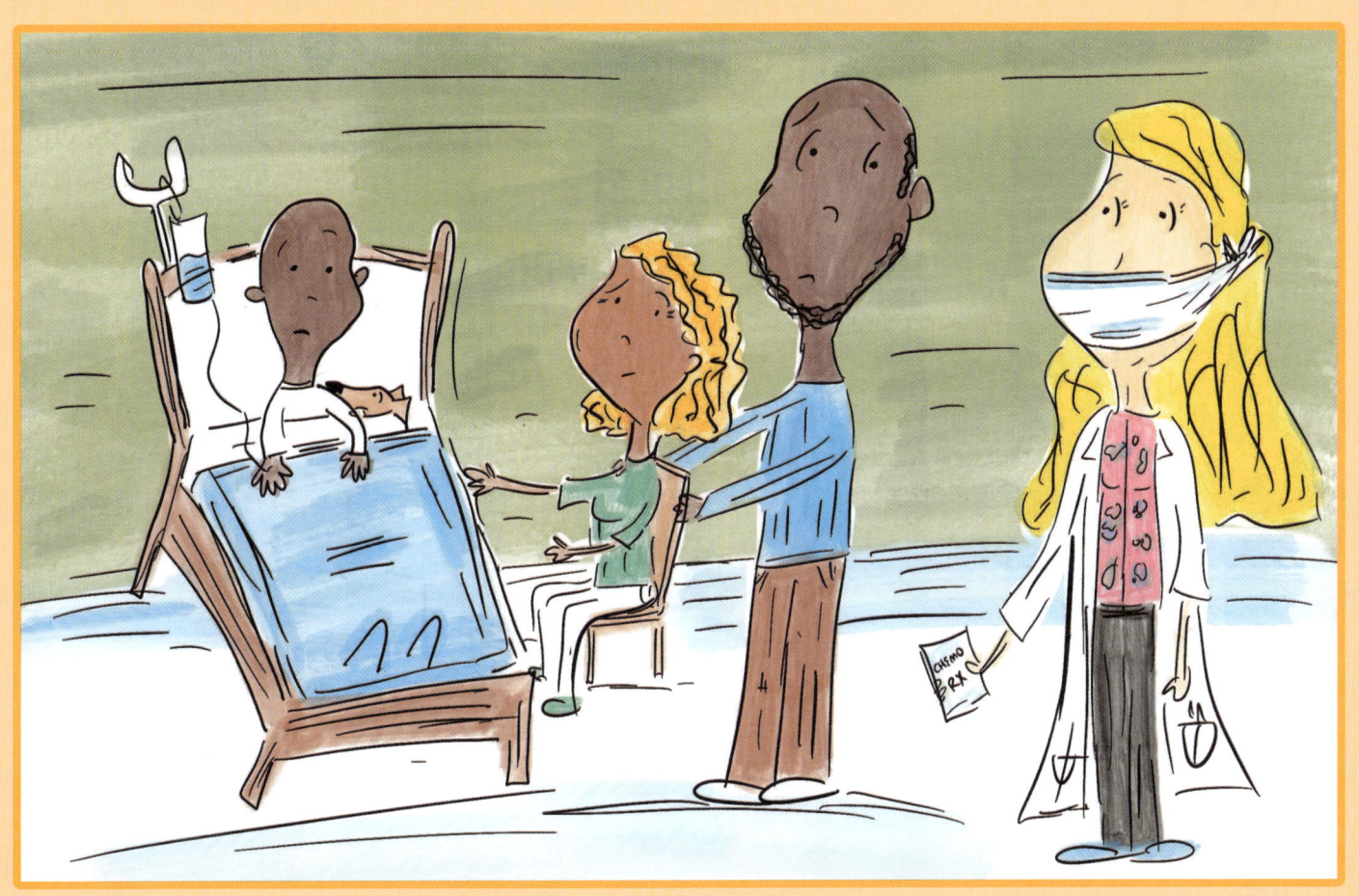

Recently I got sick and I had to go to the doctor. Turns out I had a type of cancer called leukemia. And I needed special medicine to help me get better. This scared me. And it scared my family.

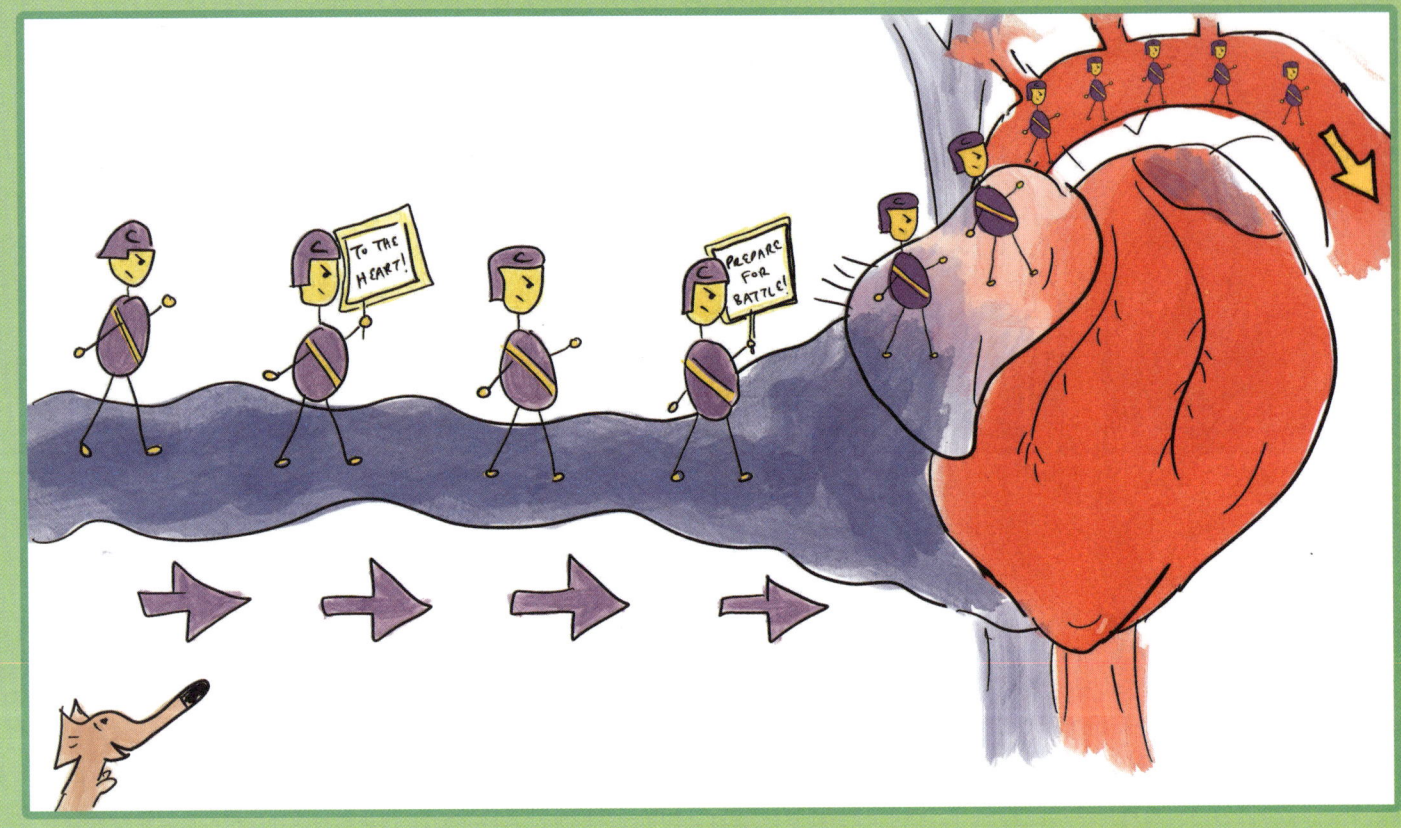

The special medicine I needed is called **chemotherapy**. It goes into veins, which are blood vessels in your body that empty into your heart. Your heart then pumps the chemotherapy all over your body so it can fight the cancer.

My chemotherapy warriors!

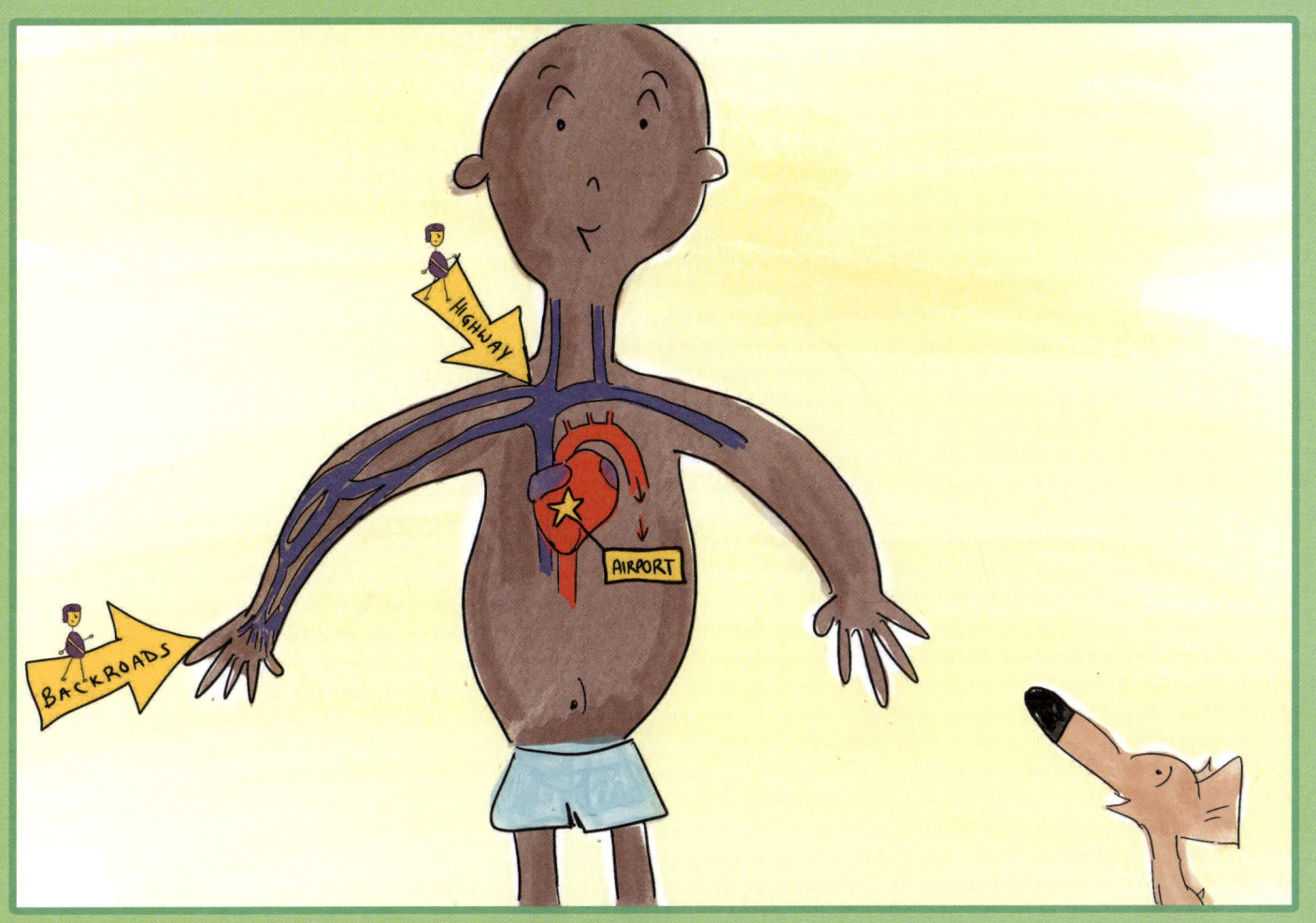

Now imagine the blood vessels in your body are like roads.
And your heart is the airport. Your little veins that run in your
arms are like the small windy back roads.
And the big veins in your neck and chest are like the big
highways that quickly enter your heart.

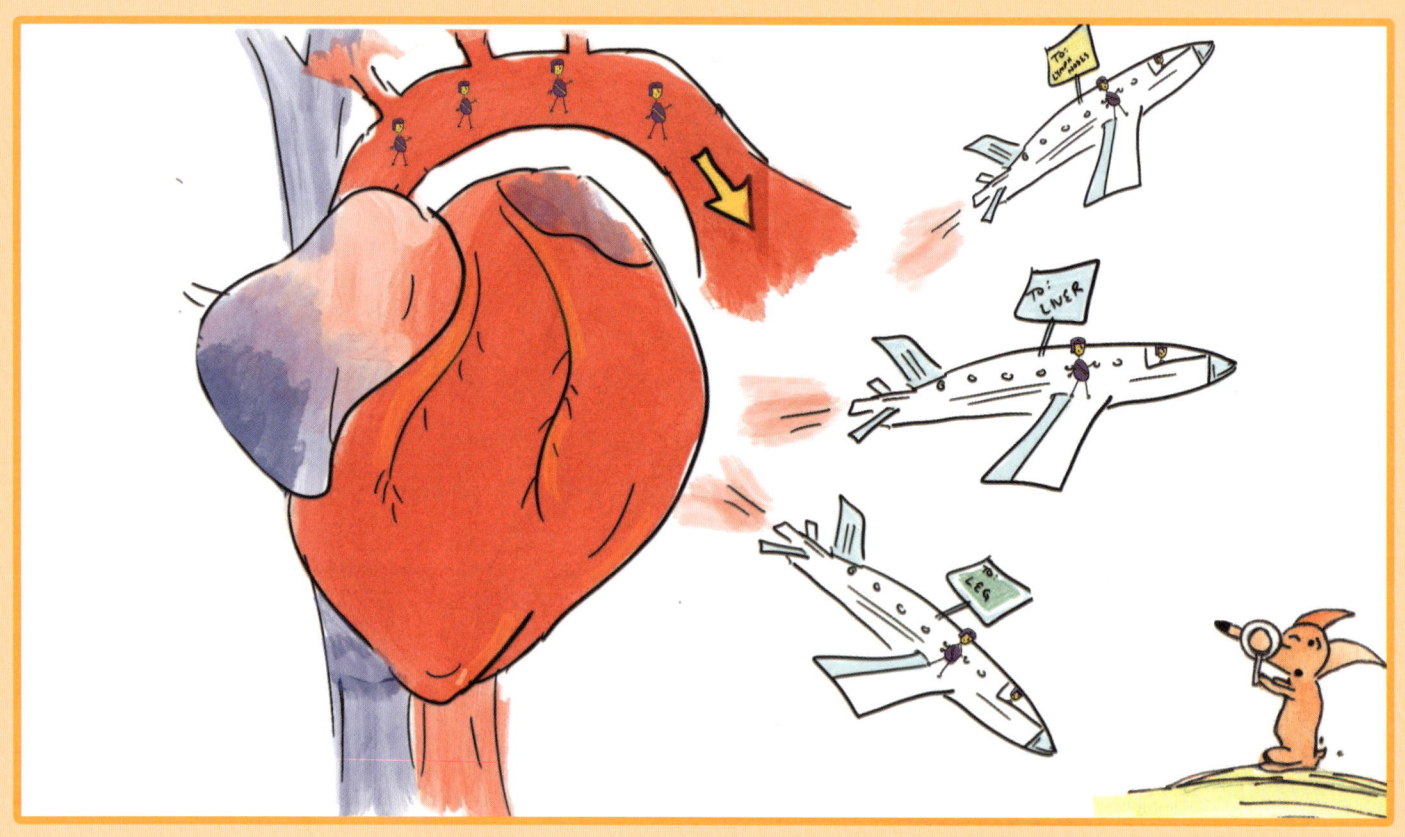

What's the best way to get the chemotherapy warriors to your heart? If the warriors take the small backroads, it will be a long time before they reach the heart. Sometimes they don't even get there because of the bumps and detours. If they take the highway, the warriors go straight to the heart. No delays!

Time to fly off to the rest of the body!

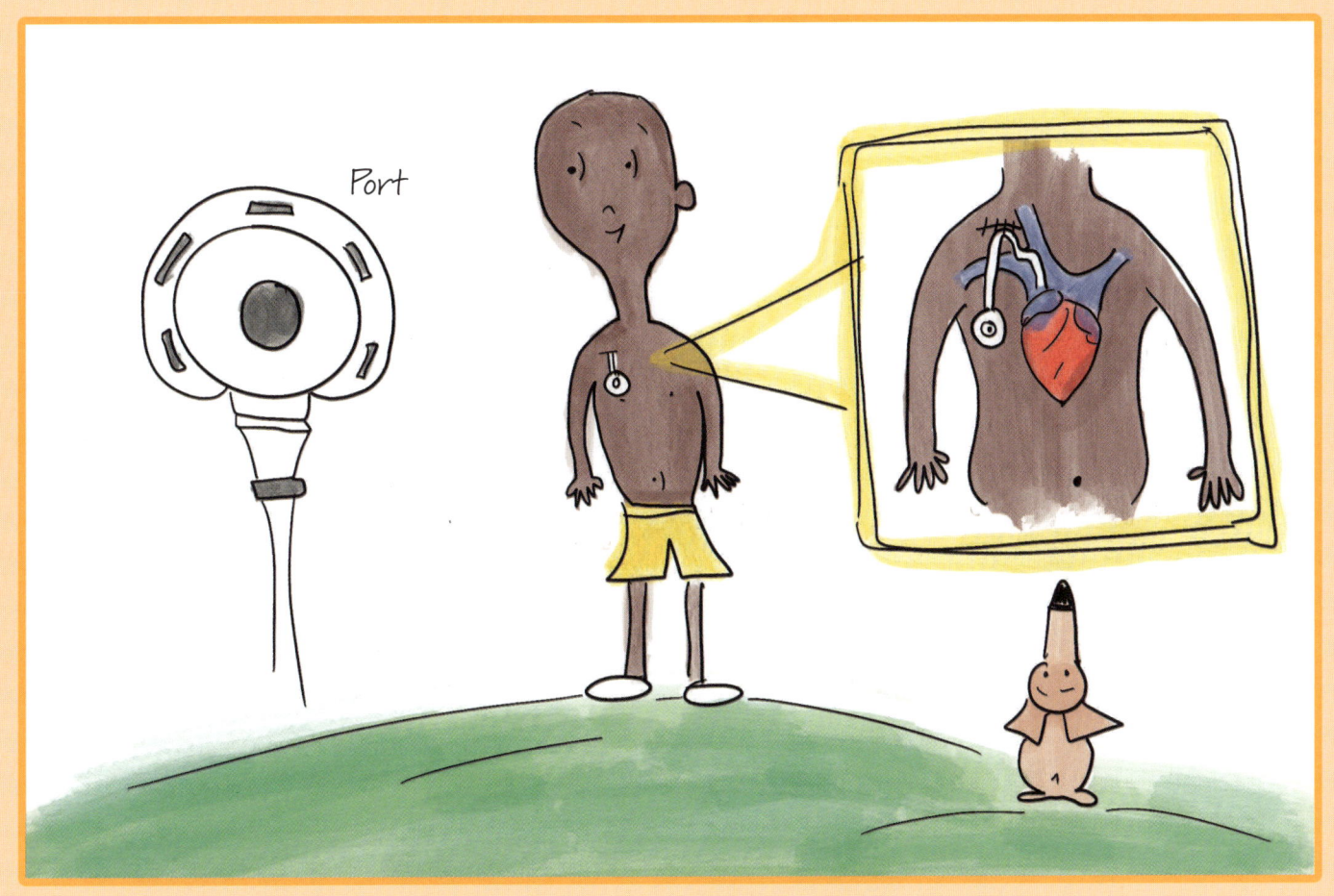

That's why I needed a **central line**. It acts as
entry ramp to the highway for my chemotherapy warriors.
The type I got is called a **port**.

There are three different kinds of central lines: 1) **Ports** (like mine!) 2) tunneled
central lines (**CVC**) and 3) peripherally inserted central catheters (**PICC**).

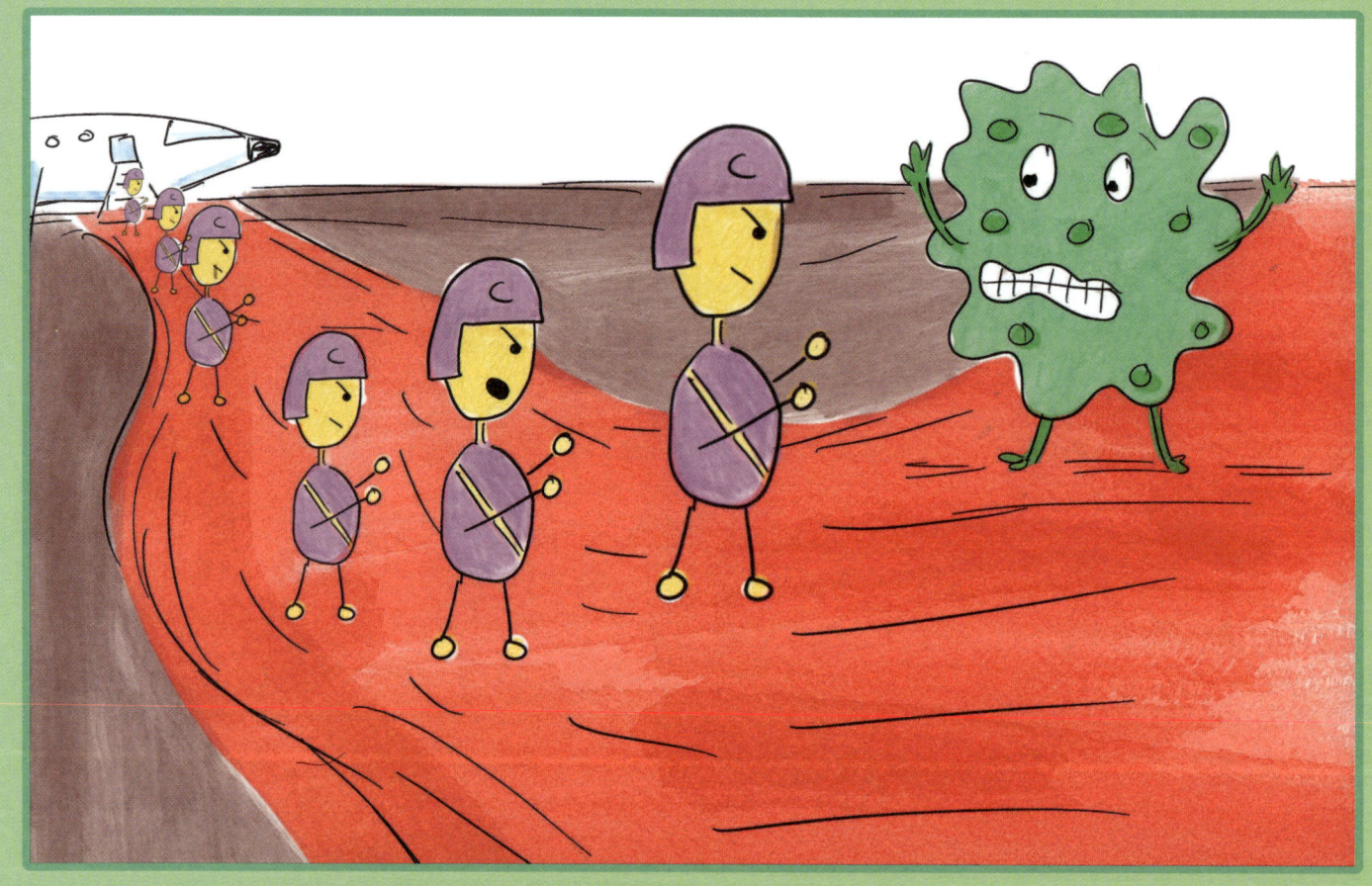

Now my chemotherapy warriors enter at my central line, go through my big vein highways, and get right to my heart! My airport heart then pumps them all over my body to fight my cancer!

Watch out cancer!

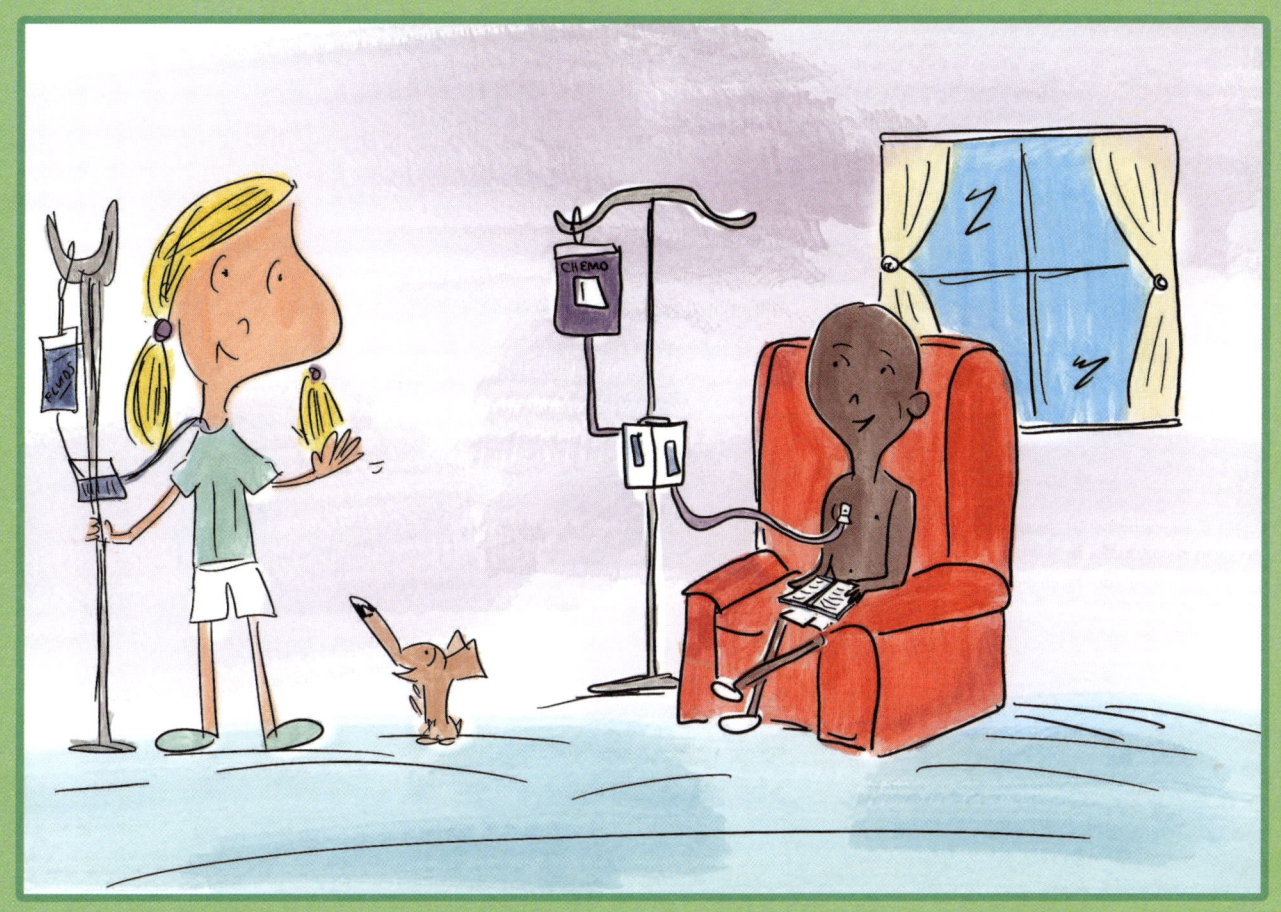

Some kids need central lines for other things besides chemotherapy. Other medicines, fluids and food to stay strong, or to take some drops of blood to test. For whatever reason, they all work the same way!

They are highways to the heart!

Facts

Airports are the best way for people and things to get to distant places - FAST! Things like medicine. Or food. Or presents for loved ones! And highways get people and things to airports quickly. And easily. Without highways or airports, people and things wouldn't get easily to places where they are needed.

This is just like the **circulatory system** in our body! Our hearts are in charge of pumping blood, oxygen, and nutrition to every cell in our bodies. Just like an airport! And just like a highway, a **central line** is a direct, FAST road to the heart. That's why it's called a 'central' line. Because it goes right to the middle of your body - your heart. It gets things that our bodies need to our heart quickly. Like medicines. Or fluids. Or food.

Check out this map to compare a real heart to the story's airport analogy!

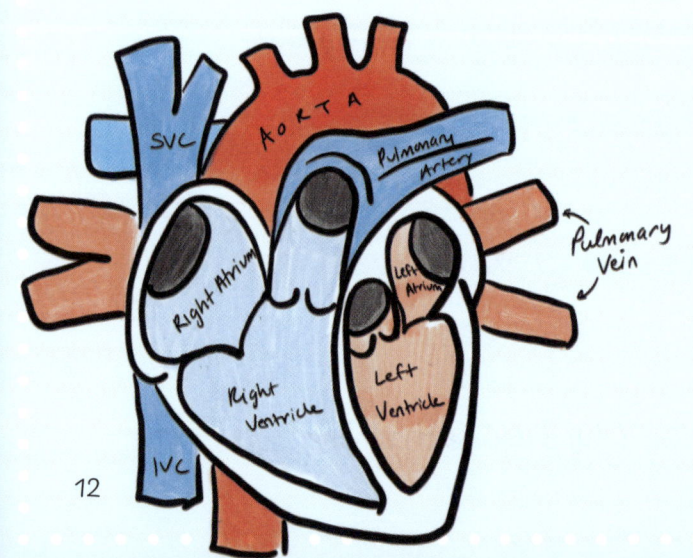
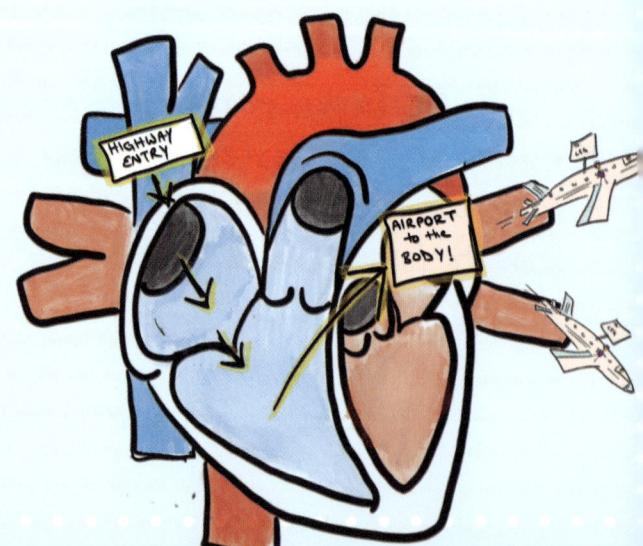

Central lines make it easy to access your blood vessels for medicines and tests.

There are three different types of central lines. **Ports, tunneled central lines** (CVC) and **peripherally inserted central catheters** (PICC lines).

All three types of lines can be used for:

- Medicine like chemotherapy
- Nutrition to keep you strong (called TPN)
- Fluids to hydrate you
- Blood draws for tests

Medicine like chemotherapy can hurt small blood vessels. Also, when you need medicine often, it hurts to get poked with needles each time. A central line lets medicine, fluids, or nutrition get directly into the large vein near your heart. This keeps your small blood vessels safe. And you don't have to get poked with needles every time.

The main differences between the three types of central lines involve:

- Placement (a procedure or at bedside)
- Where it starts/enters into your body
- How long it can stay in
- How to take care of it
- Risks / complications

Let's learn a little more about each type of central line!

Ports

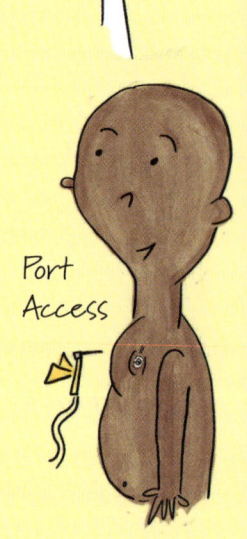

Port

Catheter

Port-a-cath (Port). That's what Anthony got in this story!
A port is a small circle (the size of a quarter) that sits under your
skin by your collarbone. There is no tubing outside of your skin.

Ports have two parts:

1) **Port** — a little container that sits like a bump under your skin. It is
   where needles are inserted. It is the size of a quarter!

2) **Catheter** — the small tube attached to the port that travels under
   your skin to the large vein near your heart

Port
Access

Ports are placed in the operating room (surgery) or in a
radiology suite (procedure room). It can stay in for **years**!

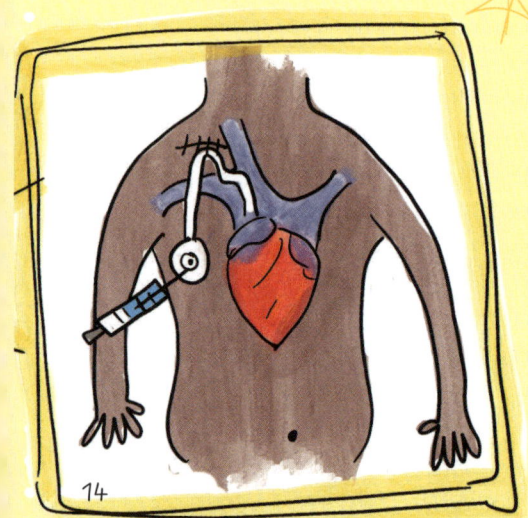

Taking care of your port:

- When your port is not being used, a dressing will
  cover it. Try your best to keep the dressing dry.
- You can still shower or swim. Just make sure the dressing is
  covered with plastic and tape. If it gets wet, replace the dressing.
- Ports need to be flushed every month with 5 mL of heparinized
  saline.
- They also need to be flushed with 10–20 mL of sterile saline
  after blood draws and medicines.
- Don't worry! Your doctor and nurse will give you specific
  instructions and teach you how to flush it!

14

CVC

Tunneled central lines (CVC) are another type of central line. This type of line starts in one of the large veins in your neck or under your collarbone and ends at your heart. It has tubing that comes out of your skin.

A CVC has two parts

1) **Catheter** – the tube that travels from the large vein in your neck or collarbone to your heart
2) **Lumens** – the ends of the catheter that you give medicine through. There are usually one or two lumens. They dangle over your skin.

A CVC is placed in the operating room (surgery) or in a radiology suite (procedure).

CVCs can stay in for **days to months**.

Taking care of your CVC:

• When your CVC is not being used, a dressing will cover it. Try your best to keep the dressing dry.
• Try to avoid tugging or pulling on your CVC. Be careful when you play!
• No swimming! You can shower/bathe with a waterproof dressing over your CVC.
• CVCs need to be flushed every day with 5 mL of heparinized saline.
• CVCs need to be flushed with 10–20 mL of sterile saline after blood draws & medicines.
• Don't worry! Your doctor and nurse will give you specific instructions and teach you how to flush it!

Catheter

Lumens

PICC

Peripherally inserted central catheter (PICC line) is the final type of central line. A PICC line starts in one of the large veins in your arms and ends at your heart. It has tubing that comes out of your skin.

PICC Catheter

Lumens

A PICC has two parts
1) **Catheter** – the tube that travels from the large arm vein to your heart
2) **Lumens** – the ends of the catheter that you give medicine through. There are usually one or two.

No surgery is needed to place a PICC line!!

It can be placed at bedside by a skilled nurse using an **ultrasound**! Or by a radiology doctor in the **interventional radiology** (IR) procedure room.

Taking care of your PICC:

 PICCs can stay in for **days to months.**

- When your PICC is not being used, a dressing will cover it. Try your best to keep the dressing dry.
- Try to avoid tugging or pulling on your PICC. Be careful when you play!
- No swimming! You can shower/bathe with a waterproof dressing over your PICC.
- PICCs need to be flushed every day with 5 mL of heparinized saline.
- PICCs need to be flushed with 10–20 mL of sterile saline after blood draws & medicines.
- Don't worry! Your doctor and nurse will give you specific instructions and teach you how to flush it!

Procedure Details

- Either a surgeon or radiologist will put a CVC or port in. A PICC line usually does not need a procedure. It is placed at bedside by a special nurse with ultrasound.
- Don't eat after midnight the night before! You can drink water 2 hours before.
- Placing the CVC or port takes about 30 minutes.
- You will be asleep during it, so you won't feel a thing.
- Your doctor uses a needle (sometimes with an ultrasound) to find your big vein and puts the catheter into it. The catheter travels through the vein right to your heart.
- This catheter will attach to the port or to your CVC lumens.
- Afterwards, you will have some purple glue over your incision or a bandage. This glue will peel off in several weeks. Do not peel if off on your own.

Risks include:

- **Pneumothorax** (a collapsed lung): There is a small risk of this happening during CVC or port placement. It happens in 1 out of 100 people. If this happens, doctors will do x-rays and watch you closely. You may need a small chest tube to help your lung fill with air again.

- **Thrombosis** (a blood clot): There is a small risk of thrombosis in either your line or your blood vessels. Based on where the clot is, you may need medicine or we may need to remove your CVC or port or PICC.

- **Infection**: There is a small risk that your line can get infected. This happens in 5 out of 100 people (ports or PICCs) and in 15 out of 100 people (CVCs). If this happens, we may need to remove it and you may need antibiotics. To stay safe from infection, only let your medical team touch your central line unless you have been told otherwise.

17

Doctor Words

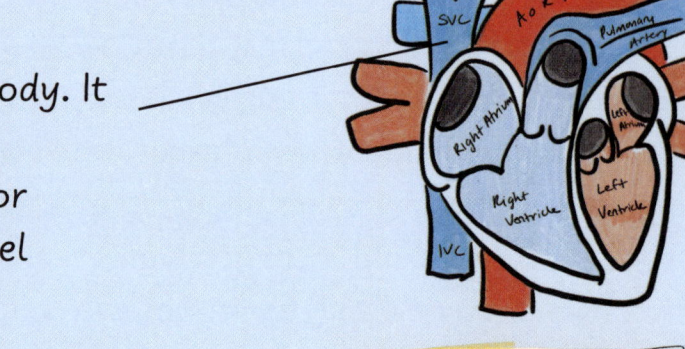

Superior vena cava (SVC): One of the biggest blood vessels in your body. It leads right into your heart. It's the highway!! Your catheter (tubing) for your port, CVC, and PICC lines travel right into it.

Catheter: a fancy word for the tubing part of your central line.

Circulatory System: a system of organs that include the heart, blood vessels, and blood. The circulatory system's job is to move blood through your body. It starts with the heart. Your heart pumps blood, oxygen, and nutrition into blood vessels. Blood vessels called arteries carry the blood to every cell in your body. Blood vessels called veins return the blood back to the heart.

OR: The operating room! It's a big special room where a surgeon puts in your port or CVC. You won't remember it. You'll be sound asleep.

Interventional Radiology (IR): a field of medicine. Doctors in IR are called **radiologists**. They may put in your port, CVC, or PICC line.

TPN: Nutrition given through a vein when you can't eat by mouth. It supplies all daily food and nutrition needs.

Anesthesia: Medicine to put you to sleep while your CVC or port is placed. When you wake up, you might be really confused and sleepy; but that's normal!

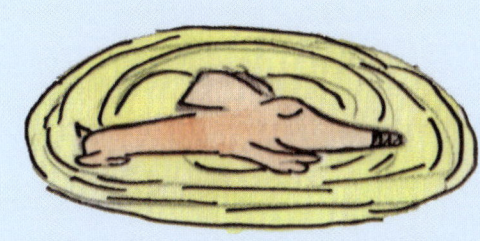

Ultrasound: A safe, painless way to look at your blood vessels. This helps your doctor place your CVC or port. It also helps a nurse or radiologist place your PICC line.

Dermabond: Purple glue that helps hold your surgery cut together. It will peel off on its own in several weeks. Don't peel it off yourself.

Steri-strips: Small, sticky bandages that help hold your surgery cut together. Some doctors like to use this instead of the purple glue. They will fall off on their own as well so try not to peel them off.

Heparin: A medicine used to help prevent your catheter (tubing) from clogging.

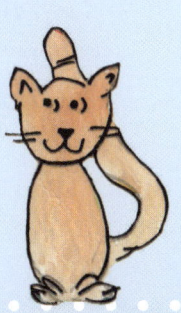

Meet the Author:
Dr. Maria Baimas-George

Maria Baimas-George MD MPH is an abdominal transplant surgeon. Inspired by her patients and mentors, she writes and illustrates books explaining medical and surgical conditions to children and their loved ones. Her goal is to create books that provide useful information to help with understanding and to offer comfort and hope.

WINNER OF THE 2021 SILVER TOUCHSTONE AWARD

Awarded for exceptional performance in patient safety, clinical outcomes, efficiency & service excellence

Please visit us online at **www.StrengthOfMyScars.com** to learn more about our team and story and see our full collection of available books.

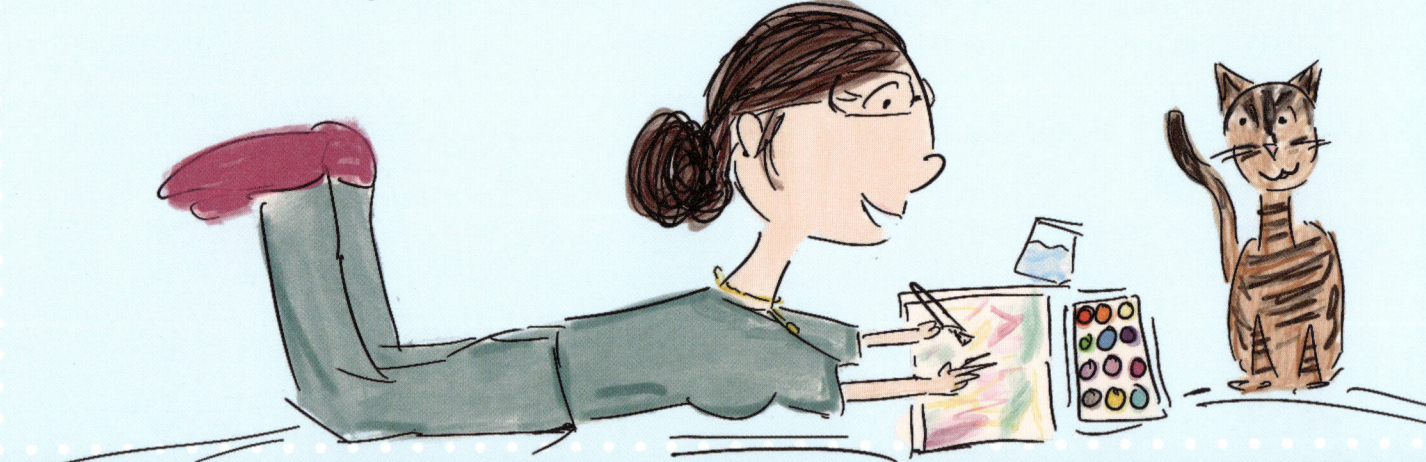